I0438214

Mercy Nurses

The making of a Mercy Nurse

By

Marlys Floyd

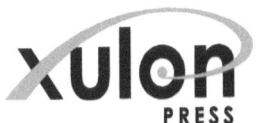

PRESS

The imprimatur for the booklet <u>Mercy Nurses: The Making of a Mercy Nurse.</u>

> Nihil Obstat:
> > Rev. Richard L. Schaefer
> > Censor Deputatus

> Imprimatur:
> > Most Rev. Jerome Hanus, O.S.B.
> > Archbishop of Dubuque

The following disclaimer about the nihil obstat and the imprimatur should be included:

The nihil obstat and imprimatur are official
Declarations that a book or pamphlet is free of
Doctrinal or moral error. No implication is
  contained
Herein that those who granted the nihil obstat
  and
Imprimatur agree with the contents, opinions, or
Statements expressed.

Original Contributors

Sister Mary Eleanor Cashman, RSM
Various Mercy School of Nursing alumni

Reviewers:
> Sister Mary Eleanor Cashman, RSM
> Mercy School of Nursing Alumni
> Health Committee Members

> Invitational Readings References:

These can be found in the Busse library, on the Mount Mercy College Campus; or in the Religious Library located in the Sacred Heart Convent.

> Holland, Sr. Mary Ildephonse. (1952) Lengthened Shadows. NY: Bookman Associates

> Mercy Through the Years Calendar. Mercy International Center.

Roth, Sr. Mary Augustine (1980) Courage and Change. IA: Stamats Communication, Inc.

Roth, Sr. Mary Augustine (1976) Written in His Hands. IA: Laurence Press Co.

Rowe, L (1992) On Call. MI Baker Book House

Ulrich, B. L. (1992) Leadership and Management According to Florence Nightingale. CT: Appleton & Lange.

Life is mostly froth and bubble.
But two things stand in stone,
Kindness in another's trouble,
Courage in your own.

- Author Unknown

The nurse's inward journey is charted by
compassion and motivated by the desire
to diminish suffering."

Florence Nightingale.

"Every person is a tree, with roots,
with leaves,
with blossoms, with fruit that change
with the seasons."

A. Costello

Chapter 1

Mercy Heritage

Mercy Heritage
(Courtesy of Sister Mary Eleanor Cashman, RSM)

<u>1831</u> The Cedar Rapids Sisters of Mercy rejoice in their foundress, Catherine Elizabeth McAuley, who established the order in Dublin, Ireland in 1831. In addition to the vows of poverty, chastity and obedience that religious normally take, the Sisters of Mercy take a fourth vow, "care of the poor, sick and uneducated." Known namely in Dublin as the "Walking Sisters" the name was given to them because of their visiting the sick in their homes and taking food to the poor.

<u>1843</u> The first Sisters of Mercy came to Pittsburgh in America upon the request of the newly appointed Bishop, James O'Connor, who was seeking Sisters "to teach the children and nurse the sick." Led by Sister Mary Francis Warde, three professed Sisters, two novices and a postulant, they left their convent Carlow, which had been established form Dublin in 1837, and began their journey to America. On November 10th they boarded the Queen of the West and after a stormy voyage came into New York's harbor. By Christmas they were in their new home-a four-story building on Penn Street. Records indicate that the very next day, "Sisters began their work of visiting the sick."

<u>1846</u> From the time their arrival in the United States, Bishop Quarter of Chicago had been urging them to send Sisters to help in his area. This request was fulfilled by Sister Francis Warde in 1846. From Chicago, sisters went to DeWitt, Iowa in 1867. Under the leadership of Sister Mary Borromeo Johnson, a hospital was built in Davenport in 1869, and she and some of the other Sisters of DeWitt transferred there. This became the motherhouse of the Sisters of Mercy.

<u>1869</u> In late March 1869, Mother Mary Borromeo responded to the request of the people of Independence, Iowa, and sent two Sisters from Davenport. Later, three Sisters came from Chicago to join Mother Mary Francis Monholland in Independence.

<u>1875</u> On a hot July day in 1875, two professed Sisters and a Novice came from Independence to Cedar Rapids at the request of Reverend Clement Lowery, to open a school in September. One month later, four additional Sisters came from Davenport to help the Sisters open St. Joseph's Academy on Third Avenue Seventh Street SE. Of special interest to us is Anna McCullough from DeWitt, who entered as a postulant in Davenport, Iowa. As a Novice she went to Independence, Iowa. She became known as Sister Mary Gertrude and was one of the foundresses of the Cedar Rapids Sisters of Mercy. The other foundress is Sister Mary Agatha Mullaney, one of the four Sisters who came from Davenport in August to help at St. Joseph's Academy.

<u>1881</u> In 1881 the Diocese of Davenport was created. Since Cedar Rapids was within the Diocese of Dubuque, the Sisters of Mercy of Cedar Rapids, Iowa, became an independent motherhouse.

<u>1964</u> The Sisters moved from St. Joseph's Academy to the Green mansion in 1906. Then the Sisters moved into the newly constructed Sacred Heart Convent, their new Motherhouse, on March 4, 1964. Dominating the building was the octagonal chapel which seat 400. Rising from the center of the tile-shingled roof was a 94-foot fleche surmounted by a metal Cross.

<u>1989</u> The Catherine McAuley Center for Women officially opened on September 1, 1989. It is designed for women who need tutoring in areas of literacy, domestic and creative arts, and personal life skills, and who also have a need for help with child care during learning sessions. Since then, a housing program for homeless single women has been added.

<u>1990</u> After much soul searching and discussion the Cedar Rapids Sisters of Mercy and the Mount Mercy College Board of Trustees made a momentous decision. The Sisters of Mercy sold part of their Motherhouse, including the Chapel, to Mount Mercy College. This was an effort to downsize the Motherhouse to meet the needs of the community and, in turn, offer space for a library and learning center. The college library, known as the Busse Center, opened on January 25, 1993. The building

totals 75,000 square feet and includes the library, computer science center, campus ministries area and the Chapel. The College Chapel, formerly the Motherhouse Chapel, stands on the highest point in Cedar Rapids and symbolizes the blending of heart, mind and spirit of individuals and communities. It was renamed "Chapel of Mercy."

1991 In July 1991, the twenty-five communities of the Sisters of Mercy in the United States joined together to form the Institute of the Sisters of Mercy of the Americas. Today the Sisters of the Cedar Rapids Regional Communities throughout the Americas continue the legacy of compassion and service established by Catherine McAuley in 1831.

1993 The Cedar Rapids Sisters of Mercy became a co-sponsor of Mercy Housing, Inc. in July, in an effort to provide affordable housing for the needy. Other co-sponsors of the agreement are Sisters of Mercy in Omaha, Nebraska, and Auburn, Alabama, and Burlingame, California, and Sisters of St. Joseph of Peace.

1994 The Sisters continue to fulfill the Direction Statement of the Institute of the Sisters of Mercy of the Americas.

Animated by the Gospel and Catherine McAuley's passion for the poor, we, the Sisters of Mercy of the Americas, are impelled to commit our lives and resources for the next four years to act in solidarity with:

The economically poor of the world, especially women and children.

Women seeking fullness of life and equality in church and society.

One another as we embrace our multi-cultural and international reality.

This commitment will impel us to develop and act from a multi-cultural, international perspective; speak with a corporate voice; work for systemic change; and call ourselves to continual conversion in our lifestyle and ministries.

July 1991

Ministries

The first Sisters of Mercy to come to Cedar Rapids set the example that continues today in responding to the needs of the times in the spirit of Catherine McAuley. Originally the Sister's ministry was principally in Iowa and Montana, with teaching, nursing and social work predominating. Today Sisters are in Florida, Iowa, Illinois, Indiana, Kansas, Minnesota, Missouri, Montana, New Mexico, Ohio, Texas, Washington, DC, West Virginia, Wisconsin, and Peru.

Sisters of Mercy from the Cedar Rapids Regional Community are missioned and serve in various ministries such as education, health care, pastoral care, social work, prayer, administration, clerical work and volunteering. Retirement is emerging as a recognized ministry. Central to all ministries is the ministry of prayer.

Reflections affirm that each of these Sisters, in her own way and in her time, has served God and humankind very well. They have followed the way of poverty, chastity, and obedience and the service of the poor, sick and uneducated.

This is a way that leads to the very heart of God. This way of life calls for a willing sacrifice of self and a dependence upon God. These special women inspire and encourage us who work with others to mirror their attitude. Jesus' ministry on earth consisted of healing and offers of wholeness always in the spirit of love. We can share in that work.

Chapter 2

Catherine McAuley

The Spirit of Mercy

Rooted in the Spirit of Mercy with Catherine McAuley as the foundress, I believe that her heart is shown in some of these lovely quotes from her writings, instruction her Sisters, and it can be used today by any of us for a guide.

"Theirs has been and is to be a Spirit of Mercy, a practical charity for Mercy is love in Action."

"Be sure you have a comfortable cup of tea for them when I am gone."

"Remember me affectionately to all. "

"Preserve union and peace. Do this and your happiness will be so great as to cause you to wonder."

"We should never falter in our confidence that God makes all things turn to the best."

"How can we teach the love of God of our own hearts are cold?"

"God never refuses grace to those who ask it."

"Show your instructions in action as much as you can."

"Now and again bestow some praise."

"Our participation in Jesus' saving mission transforms our ordinary actions as well as our joys and sorrows."

"God does not look at the action but at the spirit motivating it."

"We should never forget that as all other gifts, prayer must come from God."

"Prayer will do more than all the money in the bank of Ireland."

"It is for God we serve the poor and not for thanks."

"The great adage, 'never too old to learn,' is a great comfort to me."

"As love begets love, politeness begets politeness."

"The union which exists among you will draw down the favor and blessings of heaven."

"What can the Father refuse us, having given us His beloved Son."

"The constant interchange of prayer and service nourish one another."

"Sadness lessens the value of work performed in God's name, for God loves a cheerful giver."

"You must be cheerful and happy, animating all around you."

"The proof of love is deed."

"Above all things constant, fervent prayer."

"It is God's will that everyone called to his service be happy."

"We must cultivate the most tender devotion to the Mother of our Redeemer."

"The dignity of our Blessed lady is expressed in the one title – Mother of God."

"The comfort soon comes after a well received trial."

"Be slow to censure, and slower still to blame."

"Your conversation should be simple, pleasant and useful."

"It is Jesus Christ you love and serve with your whole heart."

"We should implore the assistance of the Blessed Virgin in all our actions."

- Catherine McAuley

Chapter 3

Spiritual and Corporal Works of Mercy

Works of Mercy

The Spiritual and Corporal works of mercy have been the source of inspiration to many people. They can guide us in our journey in mercy through the ministry of caregiving.

We affirm and acclaim our charism to be mercy. Mary, the first ecclesiastical woman, is our inspiration. Following the example of others and Catherine McAuley, we live the Spiritual and Corporal works of mercy in a spirit of hospitality of heart and servanthood.

- Mission Statement 1978

SPIRITUAL WORKS OF MERCY

Counseling the Doubtful: The caregiver is an advocate for others in health and in illness. The caregiver's behavior reflects consideration of others dignity, beliefs, values and needs.

Instruct the ignorant: Caregivers provide health education that is informational and supportive. Examples include knowledge related to medications, tests and procedures, and individual or group opportunities.

Forgiving Injuries: Health care is changing rapidly. Effective teamwork affirms the opportunity to be Mercy with others.

Comforting the Sorrowful: The Caregiver touches the hearts and lives of others, as well as her/his co-workers, in times of loss. These losses can be: biophysical such as bladder control, mobility or speech; psychosocial, such as intellectual functioning or death of a family member, friend or caregiver; environmental, such as room relocation; social isolation; and multiple losses.

Admonishing the Sinner: The caregiver has a leadership accountability to create a climate of faithfulness to the greatest of all commandments, "Love."

Praying for the living and the dead: The caregiver as an advocate to the patient must work with family to facilitate "what is sacred to this person" and initiating the meeting o the Spiritual needs of this person.

Bearing injustices patiently: Sudden, chronic, or terminal illness can be perceived as "not fair." With empathy and patience the caregiver provides comfort measures and supports the patients in their suffering.

CORPORAL WORKS OF MERCY

<u>**Giving drink to the thirsty:**</u> "Be sure that you have a comfortable cup of tea for them when I am gone," instructed Catherine McAuley foundress of the Sisters of Mercy. The caregiver extends this charisma of Mercy hospitality throughout her/his shift to patients and co-workers.

<u>**Feeding the hungry:**</u> The caregiver facilitates healthy choices in dietary needs. Patients who have special dietary needs will be given appropriate meals and supplements, and will be provided with assistive devices and timely caregiver support.

<u>**Visiting the imprisoned:**</u> Room boundaries, physical restraints, wheel chair confinement and aphasia are a few examples that impede socialization. caregivers together plan and provide meaningful, diversional activities. These can include being a friend or a companion to stimulate the heart and mind to maintain the patient's optimal quality of life.

<u>**Clothing the naked:**</u> The caregiver assists others in dressing and activities of daily living (ADL's). Respect is given to the patient's personal needs, including clothing choices and hair/nail care.

<u>**Visiting the sick:**</u> Healing focuses on disease of mind and spirit, and addresses the person on many levels. Caregivers enhance opportunities to make "ordinary time" quite "extraordinary." Examples

include sharing prayer, outdoor walks, facilitating a massage, playing cards, sharing laughter, and planning therapeutic socialization with significant friends and/or family members.

Burying the dead: Death is a process into new life. Because they are often the persons consistently present with patients, caregivers hold a unique opportunity to make this closing life event meaningful. Example include: facilitating the Sacrament of the Sick for Catholics, close friends, family and caregivers; providing physical comfort measures; enhancing personal care and death with dignity and based on the patient's preference as stated in the Advanced Directives for My health Care; and honoring the prayer vigil among companions and friends during the hours of death – honoring others religions customs in this area and carrying them out.

Sheltering the homeless: Often health centers are temporary homes and/or shelters for the ill and elderly. As a caregiver/employee, we have the unique opportunity to create a safe, comfortable environment and to be advocates for the patient's needs, preferences, and choices.

Prayer to the Holy Spirit

Come Holy Spirit – come forth from within us and help us to accept and live your gifts. Let your presence be seen through us, your love radiate from us, your power heal us. May we activate your life in each other. Thank you for your presence with us now. Let us hear the ways you speak to us. Let us learn and understand what you want us to know and do through you work – Your inspiration and each other. Amen

Some Biblical healings to inspire us as caregivers to be aware we are obeying God each day as we care lovingly for others.

God's promises of healing in the Old Testament to those who return to Him:

For I will restore you to health. Of your wounds I will heal you, says the Lord. Jeremiah 31:17

Come, let us return to the Lord for it is he who has wounded, but He will heal us. Hosea 6:1

He pardons all your iniquities. He heals all your ills. Psalms 103:3

Stricken because of their wicked way and afflicted because of their sin. Psalms 107:17

They cried to the Lord in their distress. From their straits He rescued them. Psalms 107:19

Let them make thank offerings and declare His works with shouts of joy. Psalms 107:22

Although the Lord shall smite Egypt severely, he shall heal them; they shall turn to the Lord and he shall be won over and heal them. Isaiah 19:22

Chapter 4

Healings in the Old and New Testament

The New Testament reveals to us Jesus' healings and their circumstances. Apostles and disciples of Christ continued these healings, as Jesus promised we would after his resurrection.

> Then he summoned his twelve disciples and gave them authority to expel unclean spirits and to cure sickness and disease of every kind.   Matthew 10:1

> Cure the sick, raise the dead, heal the leprous, expel demons. The gift you have received, give as a gift.   Matthew 10:8

> … cure the sick there. Say to them, 'The reign of God is at hand.'   Luke 10:9

Some of Jesus' recorded healings:

> To the centurion Jesus said, "Go home. It shall be done because you trusted." That very moment the boy got better.   Matthew 8:13

> Suddenly a leper came forward and did him homage, saying to him, "Sir, if you will to do so, you can cure me." Jesus stretched out his hand and touched him and said, "I so will it. Be cured." Immediately the man's leprosy disappeared.   Matthew 8:2-3

Jesus entered Peter's house and found Peter's mother-in-law in bed with a fever. He took her by the hand and the fever left her. She got up at once and began to wait on him.

Matthew 8:14-15

As evening drew on, they brought him many who were possessed. He expelled the spirits by a simple command and cured all who were afflicted. Matthew 8:16

When e disembarked and saw the vast throng, his heart was moved with pity, and he cured their sick. Matthew 14:14

Large crowds of people came to him bringing with them cripples, the deformed, the blind, the mute, and many others besides. They laid them at his feet and he cured them.

Matthew 15:30

...indeed, the whole crowd was trying to touch him because power went out from him which cured all. Luke 6:19

A woman with a hemorrhage of twelve years' duration, incurable at any doctor hands, came up behind him and touched the tassel on his cloak. Immediately her bleeding stopped.

Luke 8:43-44

Some of the disciples healings in the name of Jesus:

> Act 3:6-7 Then Peter said: "I have neither silver nor gold, but what I have I give you! In the name of Jesus Christ, the Nazorean, walk!" Then Peter took him by the right hand and pulled him up. Immediately the beggar's feet and ankles became strong.

This miracle symbolized the saving power of Jesus Christ.

I Peter 2:24 In his own body he brought your sins to the cross, so that all of us, dead to sin, could live in accord with God's will. By his wounds, you were healed.

Act 5:16 Crowds from the towns around Jerusalem would gather, too, bringing their sick and those who were troubled by unclean spirits, all of whom were cured.

Acts 8:7-8 There were many who had unclean spirits, which came out shrieking loudly. Many others were paralytics or cripples, and these were cured. The rejoicing in that town rose to fever pitch.

Acts 9:34-35 Peter said to him, "Aeneas, Jesus Christ cures you! Get up and make your bed." The man got up at once. All the inhabitants of Lydda and Sharon, upon seeing him, were converted to the Lord.

Chapter 5

Our calling to the healing ministry

Yes, God so loved the

World that he gave

His only Son,

That whoever believes in

Him may not die

But have eternal life.

John 3:16

The basis for the Catholic Sacrament of healing is in this scripture:

Is there anyone sick among you? He Should ask for the presbyters of the Church. They in turn are to pray over Him, anointing him with oil in the Name (of the Lord). This prayer uttered in faith Will reclaim the one who is ill, and the Lord will restore him to health. If he has Committed any sins, forgiveness will be His. James 5:14-15

The Chronically or acutely ill Catholic should receive this sacrament. Let us all continue to conse-crate our lives and calling to Jesus' saving mission here on Earth and we will find our ordinary actions transformed into great works.

We will bring souls and bodies to the Lord for His forgiveness and healing and bring honor to Jesus.

Remember...
You are special...
You are called.

You are called to ministry.
You are a caregiver.

More importantly, you have been entrusted to offer significant contributions to the quality of life and health of those for whom you care. You are significant in their journey toward healing and wholeness and salvation.

Chapter 6

"wise quotes to learn and to live by from famous and holy people and the scriptures."

"This day I choose to brighten the journey of those around me."   - Author Unknown

"To ease another's heartache, is to forget one's own."   - Abraham Lincoln

"It is tranquil people who accomplish much."-   Henry David Thoreau

"Faith is nothing else but a right understanding of our being trusting, and allowing things to be." -   Julian of Norwich

"Courage is an inner resolution to go forward despite obstacles." - Martin Luther King, Sr.

"You are God's work of art."
-St. Paul, Ephesians 2:10
"What I am to be, I am now becoming."
                    - Author unknown

"The best way to know God is to love many things."   - Vincent Van Gogh

"Give what you have to someone. It may be better than you dare to think."
            - Henry Wadsworth Longfellow

"Just because the message may never be received does not mean it is not worth sending."   - Sigaki

"Compassion is to stand with someone through their pain."   - Henri Nouwen

"A good laugh is sunshine in a house."
                              - Wm Makepence Thackeray

"The Patient one shows much good sense."
                              - Proverbs 14:29

"A glad heart lights up the face…"
                              - Proverbs 15:13

"A cheerful glance brings joy to the heart."
                              - Proverbs 15:30

"Wisdom has built herself a house…."
                              - Proverbs 9:1

"Growth does not cease to be painful at any age."   - Mary Sarton

"Since I committed myself to others, nothing but the impossible has happened."
                              - R. Buckminster Fuller

"Become an expert in the art of discovering the good in every person."
                              - Dom Helder Camero

"If it were not for hope, the heart would break."   - English proverb

"Learn day by day to broaden your horizons."   - Ethel Barrymore

"We must always have old memories and young hopes."   - Arlene Houssage

"Whatever you are from nature, keep to it; never desert your own line of talent."
                                   - Sydney Smith

"To effect the quality of a day is the highest of arts."   - Henri David Thoreau

"A cheerful heart is good medicine, but a down spirit dries up the bones."
                                   - Proverbs 17-22

"There is always someone whose needs are greater than my own." -Author unknown

"Gray hair is a crown of glory; it is gained by virtuous living."   - Proverbs 16:31

"In the evening of this life we will be judged on love."   - Catherine of Sienna

"Christ's Sandals"

Lord, were those sandals thrown away, or do
you have them still?
The ones that Jesus wore that night he climbed
up Calvary's Hill?

They probably were torn to shreds because
the road was steep –
And spattered, too, with his own blood from
stones that cut His feet.

And yet, I'd like to have them, Lord – I'd
give them to my nurse.
She's doing things that Christ would do if He
were here on Earth.

She comforts those who are in pain, she wipes
their tears away.
Her hand upon a fevered brow cools like an
ocean spray....

Her smile is like tonic, tonic Lord; refreshing
as the rain, it causes hearts to pulsate, beat
and throb in every vein.

My nurse just walked into the room, her
countenance is sweet –
Well, bless her heart, she has them, Lord –
Christ's sandals on her feet!

"In appreciation for all you do."

- Author Unknown

Note to me from Reverend Richard Schaefer:

"I want to thank Marlys for the "Christ's Sandals" item that ends this booklet. I gave a copy of it to three Mercy Hospital nurses who were especially helpful to my Mother as she died in Mercy Hospital. My family and I were especially blessed to have been able to give this meditation to those nurses (one of whom was named "Angelica"). The nurses cried and said they would always cherish this gift.

I know this booklet will do much good in the world. But, to my mind, if it only did that good to our family and me and my mother and the nurses, that would be a wonderful contribution. Indeed, Marlys was wearing Christ's Sandals in writing this book in more ways than one."

This really meant a lot to me, just to know I have helped someone before I really even got it completed. What a blessing I hope this will be to many other readers, family members, patients or health care providers.

Marlys